# OUTDOOR SURVIVAL

*The Ultimate Outdoor Survival Guide for Staying Alive and Surviving In The Wilderness*

## Gavin Williams

**Medical Disclaimer:** This book does not contain any medical advice. The ideas and suggestions contained in this book are not intended as a substitute for consulting with your doctor. All matters regarding your health require medical supervision.

## ERRORS

Please contact me if you find any errors.

My publisher and I have taken every effort to ensure the quality and correctness of this book. However, after going over the book draft time and again, we sometimes don't see the forest for the trees anymore.

If you notice any errors, I would really appreciate it if you could contact me directly before taking any other action. This allows me to quickly fix it.

**Errors**: errors@semsoli.com

## REVIEWS

Reviews and feedback help improve this book and the author.

If you enjoy this book, I would greatly appreciate it if you were able to take a few moments to share your opinion and post a review online.

# SHTF
## PREPPING.

### THE PROVEN INSIDER SECRETS FOR SURVIVAL, DOOMSDAY AND DISASTER PREPAREDNESS

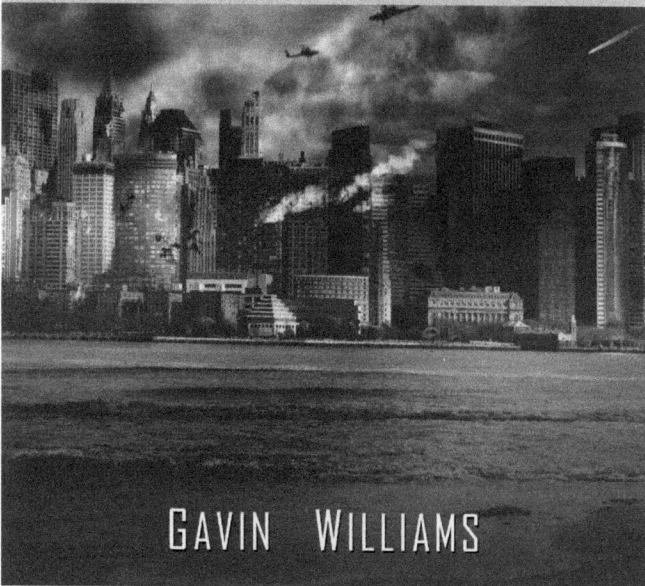

#### GAVIN WILLIAMS

# TABLE OF CONTENTS

# INTRODUCTION

I want to thank you and congratulate you for buying this book 'Survival: The Ultimate Outdoor Survival Guide for Staying Alive and Surviving In The Wilderness'.

This book has lots of actionable information on how to prep to survive in the wilderness or a dangerous situation.

The phrase "it's a jungle out there" is more relevant to the world today than it ever was before. Some people are too scared to admit this is the case. However, just look at how things have shaped up over the decades.

Terrorist attacks have become more and more prevalent. First Al Qaeda, now ISIS. Their teachings and beliefs only seem to have become more radical, with recorded beheadings making the rounds more than ever.

That is not all; with global warming becoming a bigger problem each day, it only looks like a matter of time before hurricanes and such kind becomes normal fair.

How do you stave off a natural disaster coming at you? What about wars? It would be naïve to believe that if a third world war were to come about, it would take the pattern of the previous two world wars. Weapons have evolved to a frankly terrifying point. Nations have stockpiles of nuclear weaponry these days; weaponry so devastating that it would take tens of thousands of years for the world to heal if they were ever used.

Moreover, too many people have guns in today's world, especially in the US. It is much more probable for an all-out war to break out today than at any other point in history. Looking at all these factors, it makes sense to prep yourself for survival. If all hell were to break loose, and this isn't a stretch by any means, only those who have trained and prepared for this situation will actually survive.

This book will teach you exactly how to increase your odds of survival.

Here is what we will discuss:

- **Chapter 1 – The Survival Rules of Three:** If you are going to survive in the wilderness, at a bare minimum you need to be familiar with the Survival Rules of Three. According to these rules, you cannot survive three minutes without air, three hours without shelter, three days without water, three weeks without food and three months without hope.

- **Chapter 2 – The Mindset Of A Survivor**: More important than anything else when trying to survive is having the right mindset. Given the circumstances, you can have all the right tools, food and water you need to live for a while. But if you don't have the will to live, you are not going to last long.

- **Chapter 3 – How To Prepare Your Survival Kit**: Preparing a survival kit is very important. Having such a kit will simplify food, clothing and shelter issues. You will learn some first and second-tier tools that you must include in your kit if you want to survive long-term.

- **Chapter 4 – How To Make A Base Camp In The Wilderness**: Finding or building a basic shelter should be a higher priority than finding water or food. Your body temperature can drop or increase rapidly without proper shelter. In this chapter, you will learn how to choose and prepare the right location for your shelter, and how to make your shelter.

- **Chapter 5 – How To Find Water**: Water is crucial for survival. You cannot survive without it for more than a few days. In this chapter, you will learn how to find water in the wilderness.

find food. In this chapter, you will learn how you can prevent starvation by stocking foods, foraging, hunting, and setting traps.

- **Chapter 10 – How To Preserve Food**: As with water, you will want to preserve some food after you have gone through the trouble of finding and cooking it. In this chapter, you will learn the basics of food preservation.

- **Chapter 11 – How To Defend Yourself**: If you have followed along so far, you will now know how to keep your head cool in the wild, create a base camp, how to make a fire, how to find water and food, and how to preserve both. With all of this in place, you will be able to survive in the wild for a long time. However, the one thing that can threaten your survival is other people and wild animals. This means you ought to find ways of defending yourself when situation demands. In this chapter, you will learn how to do so by improvising your weaponry and mastering a number of hands-on self-defense techniques.

- **Chapter 12 – How To Apply First Aid**: Regardless of how much you prepare, chances are you will still get hurt when attacked in the wild. In that case, having first aid skills can make your life a lot smoother. In this chapter, you will learn the basics of first aid, how to prepare your first aid kit, and how to maintain a survivor's mindset when you or a loved one are hurt.

- **Conclusion**: In the final chapter, we will wrap things up. After reading this book, it is time to implement the survival hacks you have learned. True mastery comes from practice!

I hope you are excited! Let's begin.

# 1. THE SURVIVAL RULES OF THREE

If you are going to survive in the wilderness, at a bare minimum you need to be familiar with the Survival Rules of Three. This is an old and well-known rule that is said to originate from the Survival, Evasion, Resistance and Escape (SERE) program that is used in the U.S. military.

According to the Survival Rules of Three, you cannot survive:

- Three minutes without air
- Three hours without shelter
- Three days without water
- Three weeks without food
- Three months without hope

***

## Three Minutes Without Air

Safety comes first. Your body cannot go without oxygen for more than three minutes. If you have every tried to count how long you can hold your breath under water, you know what I am talking about. If you cannot breathe for more than three minutes, you will likely lose consciousness. And unless the circumstances change, you will die shortly after.

The moments immediately following a disaster are the most crucial for your survival. You and your loved ones will likely experience panic, shock and fear. But this is why you prepare for surviving a disaster: so you know what to do when it hits. And the first thing you need to ensure is that you can breathe.

\*\*\*

## Three Hours Without Shelter

Next up is finding shelter, to regulate your body temperature. This is even more important in harsher conditions. If you cannot find protection from the elements in the hours after a disaster strikes, you run the risk of dying due to overheating (hyperthermia) or undercooling (hypothermia).

Look for shelter first, and only start thinking about long-term survival after you have found it.

\*\*\*

## Three Days Without Water

The next thing the body needs most after oxygen is water.

14

The body of an average adult consists for 50 to 65% of water, and for babies it is even 75%. On average, and depending on the temperature outdoors, you can do without water for three days. If it is warm, you will need water sooner. If it is cooler, you will be able to last a bit longer.

In any case, finding water should be your number one priority. Water does so much more than simply ending your thirst. Ever wondered why you are thirsty in the first place? Because water does so many wonderful things for your health:

☐ Allows the cells of your body to grow and survive
☐ Helps to digest and metabolize food
☐ Helps to deliver oxygen throughout the body

And that is just the tip of the iceberg. Water is like the oil in a car engine. Without it, the whole thing just falls apart.

Dehydration causes your heart rate and breathing to become more rapid, you will get headaches, become dizzy, and ultimately you will lose consciousness and die.

Therefore, after you have found shelter, make sure you find water next.

***

## Three Weeks Without Food

With enough water, you will be able to survive for a few weeks. Look for example at prisoners that go on hunger strike. A famous example is that of Mahatma Gandhi, the Indian political leader who led India to independence from British rule, who survived a twenty-one-day hunger strike.

However, the longer you go without food, the weaker you will become. And the weaker you are, the harder it will be to find food. So as soon as you find water, go search for things to eat.

\*\*\*

## Three Months Without Hope

All the skills, tools and techniques in the world cannot help you survive if you do not have the will to live.

This is wonderfully illustrated in the movie 'The Road', in which Charlize Theron plays Viggo Mortensen's wife in a post-apocalyptic world. She cannot handle the constant fear of being raped, eaten by cannibals and getting killed. Whereas her husband clings to his hope for a better future for them and their son, she ultimately gives up all hope and walks off into the dark, to a certain death…

In order to survive, you need to have hope for a better future.

*\*\*\**

When disaster strikes, you need to know these Survival Rules of Three more than anything else. They are easy to remember, so you are best off memorizing them. As a back-up, you may want to write them on a small piece of paper that you keep in your wallet, so you have them readily available when you really need them.

# 2. THE MINDSET OF A SURVIVOR

Before anything, you need to prepare your mind by developing a survival mindset because without it, everything else you will be learning will be all foreign concepts that you cannot relate with. That's exactly what this chapter is about. Let's begin!

What is a survivor focused on?

Is it in his interest to be comfortable? Sure enough, this is the case and yet, this is not his primary objective. His primary objective is to survive.

To survive is to simply stay alive. To stay alive means just that – stay alive regardless of how pleasant or unpleasant the conditions are. You can be as uncomfortable as uncomfortable goes and still stay alive. You can live on food you do not necessarily like and stay alive. You can survive on meager rations if it calls for it, even though you would like it better if you were to eat to your fill. You can survive in survival shelters and not necessarily have to have a proper home to live in.

***

## The Survivor's Mindset

Survival doesn't have a lot to do with being comfortable or even being happy. These are trivial elements. It has everything to do with staying alive. Think of Robert Tininenko surviving on a handful of sea water-soaked peas and a sip of water per day when he was stranded at sea. He lost over 30 pounds and yet he lived through those 72 days in hell. He wasn't comfortable in any sense. But he survived, and that is what's most important.

You need to embrace a different mindset – a survivor's mindset. This is a mindset that prioritizes staying alive and making the necessary sacrifices it takes for you to stay alive over everything else. It embraces toughness and a will to grind on when everything is falling apart all around you.

***

## What Is A Survivor's Mindset

Reality TV has no place in a survivor's mind. If anything, all TV has no place in a survivor's mind. TV mostly only provides entertainment. Off the grid, entertainment is not a priority. The likes of "Keeping up with the Kardashians" will have to die a deserved death in your head. Downing beers by the grill, while certainly a desirable option, must be relegated as it should. A survivor has no patience for anything that does not contribute to his survival, no matter if it is a luxury that makes him feel good.

A survivor will live off the grid if that is the most viable way to stay alive. When disaster strikes and things go south, you can bet living off the grid will present the best chance of survival. He or she will think nothing of making the necessary sacrifices it takes to live off grid. So what if he will not enjoy the luxury of having his shirts pressed or his bread toasted?

Poon Lim survived for 133 days in the sea with nothing more than a four-by-four makeshift raft. He had no shirt, let alone a pressed shirt every morning. 133 days is nearly half a year (four months and some days on top). He had no tools, so he tore off a piece of metal from his raft and sharpened it until it could cut through meat. He had no water and no food, so he found his drink by killing off sea gulls and drinking their blood. He would use himself as bait for sharks then catch them and eat their meat. It can't have been easy to take down seagulls on a small sized floating rig. It must have been as hard as it gets to actually kill a shark, with depleted strength reserves. And Poon Lim was never big or strong anyway, even when he was at his healthiest.

## How You Can Adopt A Survivor's Mindset

This is what we call a survivor's mindset; a mindset that is intent on staying alive; a mindset that ruthlessly takes out anything that does not regard his survival as sacred. A survivor prioritizes staying alive over everything else, regardless of the comforts he has to sacrifice. Even more so, he cultivates and maintains an iron will to stay alive.

You cannot afford to panic, for with panic comes the death of clear thought. Without clear thought, it becomes almost impossible to plan out your survival or even go through with whatever plans you have laid down. There is always light at the end of the tunnel, for this is one of the hard laws of nature. But before you can sight this light, you need to do all it takes to stay alive as hard and uncomfortable as it may be.

This is the survivor's mindset. Is this something you can do? Well, certainly it is. Because unless you value your survival, everything else we will learn in this book will amount to nothing!

With that information in mind, the first thing you ought to start doing is preparing a survival kit, as this can improve your odds of survival when disaster strikes. Let's learn how to go about that next.

# 3. HOW TO PREPARE YOUR SURVIVAL KIT

It helps to be set up for survival when disaster finally strikes. One of the best ways to set yourself up for survival is to have a proper survival kit. A survival kit does just that – it helps you to survive. In other words, it puts you in a better position to stay alive.

A survival kit will simplify food, clothing and shelter issues, which are the most essential needs a human being has.

The best survival kits abandon the spectacular for the functional. A survival kit will involve some of the most basic tools you will ever see and yet, they will make a world of difference when you are off-grid and have to improvise to live.

Here are some things you need so as to assemble a basic survival kit.

***

# The First-Tier Tools

These are the absolute most important tools to have. In fact, if you were to sacrifice all else in your survival kit, these are the tools you would preserve:

- **Folding knife**: This one is the most essential. Ask anyone who has been in a survival situation and he/she will tell you a folding knife is invaluable. You can cut off strips of bark or plants to eat, sharpen sticks to help you hunt, cut off strips of clothing to make bandages for cuts and so forth – there are endless possibilities on the stuff you can do with a proper folding knife.

- **Firestarter**: This is a strong no. 2. Fire is always important for survival. Well, if you are a smoker, don't even think that your BIC lighter is enough to survive. While still helpful, a lighter's fuel will run out swiftly. When a lighter gets wet, it will give you all sorts of hell before you can get it to light. Matches are even worse than lighters. Firesteel fire starters are the best kind for survival.

- **Cordage**: This one is used for lashings, bowstrings, snares, fishing lines, nets, trap triggers, you name it. It is always a good idea to have this on you at all times (e.g. paracord), even though it is not all that hard to make some from natural material.

***

## The Second-Tier Tools

While these are not as essential as the first-tier tools, they are still very essential in their own right and make life a lot more tolerable.

- **Compass**: Preferably, you should have a full-sized compass. A compass will give you an idea of where you are and help you travel.

- **Fixed knife**: This is a non-folding knife. A heavy-duty knife is best, especially one that can take a pounding and slicing through all sorts of things.

- **Water container**: Preferably a collapsible one that is light.

- **Water**: You can never carry enough water. However, carrying too much of it may hamper your movement and put your survival in danger. Nevertheless, it is sensible to bring some with you.

- **Water purifying kit**: Iodine crystal kits are best. Since you might run out of the water you have carried eventually, it helps to have this one handy.

- **Flashlight**: You may need to work at night, travel at night, forage for food or even hunt. A flashlight will make all of these things easier.

- **First Aid kit**: It should at the very least include tweezers, dressing agents, aspirin, antihistamine, wipes, bandages and gauze.

- **Signal mirror**: While any mirror will do for a signal mirror, custom made signal mirrors are best as they have a hole in the center that helps you better aim reflected light.

- **Food**: Canned food is best, as well as food that can stay good for a long time without spoiling.

***

When disaster strikes, you will need to understand how to create a structure where you will operate from; think of it as a base camp. Let's learn how to go about it next.

# 4. HOW TO MAKE A BASE CAMP IN THE WILDERNESS

Your warmth MUST be your #1 priority because without a synchronized body temperature (too cold or too hot), you are likely to die of hypothermia (undercooling) or hyperthermia (overheating). Therefore, you must set up shelter to keep yourself safe from the elements.

Here, you will learn the basics of making a base camp in the wilderness in a step-by-step format:

1. Choose a Location
2. Prepare the Location and Gather Necessary Materials
3. Make Your Shelter
4. Where to do Number Two

\*\*\*

## Choose a Location

The best type of location will be a semi-level one with lots of fallen debris nearby (think leaves, twigs, branches and the sort).

A tree, rock face, boulder or any large object will do for your shelter's base. It must be tall enough for you to crouch behind and wide enough for you to rest against comfortably. The other thing to do is to ensure that your location is not in such a low position that run-off may accumulate in the case of rain.

Make sure it is clear of roots and large rocks. If you can find a ditch, by all means pitch, camp in it. Ditches are great for keeping you out of the wind's way. However, if it rains, a ditch is worse than a cleared patch of ground. If you suspect it is going to rain, avoid ditches.

You will have to identify a source of water near your location. A game trail nearby is a welcome thing as well.

Also, ensure to decide the direction that your door will face even before you build anything. By default, your door will be by the sturdy tree. If you can, ensure the door faces downhill. However, it is more important to ensure that the door faces away from the wind.

\*\*\*

## Prepare the Location and Gather Necessary Materials

Clear the debris from your location. Do not dispose of it though; gather debris of different sizes.

The larger sized debris will be used as structural elements and the smaller-sized debris will be handy for insulation. You will require a large log that has a forked end (for your base camp's frame). Make sure that the sticks and logs are not rotten; rotten material makes for shaky structures.

Arrange your sticks so that you have piles of different sizes. You should also collect as many pine needles, leaves and grasses as you can (for ground insulation).

***

## Make Your Shelter

Take the large log with the forked end and lean it so that the forked end leans against the tree. Ensure that this first part of your structure is as sound as can be, as this will be the foundation of your shelter.

Lean the rest of your sticks and logs against the log.
For best results, cover the two sides completely as this will make your shelter better.
Start by leaning the large sticks and move on to the medium sized sticks and small ones.

The small sticks should be used to fill the inevitable gaps between the larger and medium sized sticks.

Now place your grasses and pine needles on the ground inside your shelter for insulation.

\*\*\*

## Where To Do Number Two?

Unlike a regular home, you do not want to build a toilet in your shelter. You can't just flush things down the sewer.

So where do you go, *when* you have to go?

If you have to pee, you can simply go into the woods and do your thing. Because of the way they are built, men have it a bit easier than women, but it shouldn't really be an issue for both. Hygiene is very important though: make sure you don't pee anywhere where the urine can mix with your drinking water. Although urine is relatively sterile, you wouldn't want it in your coffee, would you?

If you have to do a number two, you will need to get a bit more creative. If you are on your own, you may choose to just walk 5 – 10 minutes away from your shelter and do your thing on the ground. But if there's two of you, or even more, this is not your best option. All that human waste will start to smell pretty badly.

Alternatively, you can build a latrine, which resembles a normal toilet. However, that too will become quite smelly. I recommend digging a cat hole. This is a hole that is 6 to 8 inches deep and is dug in the ground with a small trowel. I still suggest you keep some distance from your shelter, for reasons of hygiene. Ideally, you will want to dig a cat hole in bacteria rich soil, which will speed up the waste breakdown. If you have any toilet paper, bury it along with your waste, or burn it. When you are finished, fill up the hole.

What if you don't have any toilet paper? A good alternative are coffee filters, or pages from a phonebook.

If you only have access to natural alternatives, try using leaves. Be careful though: you don't want to use any leaves that can irritate your skin. So do a little test run first. You can also try moss collected from fallen logs or trees, or corn husks.

Finally, always wash your hands after doing your business. If pathogens carried in feces make their way back into the body, they can cause diseases. And you can't just call your doctor for an appointment when you are living in the woods...

***

Having found a good location and set up your 'base camp', your next order of business is to find water (yes, before you can even think of food!).

# 5. HOW TO FIND WATER

Water is extremely important for survival.

Think of this for a second: you can last for up to three weeks without eating. Granted; you will be weak, but you will stay alive. But, on average, you cannot go for more than three days without water. This is why people who fast are recommended to at least drink water. You will need to have a constant water supply.

If you can, make sure you have water with you at all times. However, your water supply will not last forever. If that happens, how do you go about finding water in the wilderness when your supply is gone?

Here are the six steps to finding water in the wilderness:

1. Listen for water sources
2. Look for animal tracks
3. Move downhill
4. Find insects
5. Find damp or muddy soil
6. Collect rainwater

***

## Listen For Water Sources

Listening for water sources is the most basic step. Simply stand quietly and listen as it will be hard to hear a stream or river when you are busy crushing twigs underfoot.
Stand still for five minutes at a time and pay attention to anything that sounds like a stream. Because of the sounds they make, streams and rivers are about the easiest water sources to find.

They are some of the safest as well, as the steady flow makes it hard for algae and bacteria to grow.

***

## Look For Animal Tracks

Look for animal tracks that are converging. Well, solitary animal tracks will rarely mean much but if you notice converging animal tracks, chances are high that there is a watering place somewhere. Search that immediate area and you may find water.

***

# Move Downhill

If you can neither notice converging tracks nor hear water, the next best thing is to move into a rocky crevice or valley.

Rainwater naturally drains downward, as will river water. Chances are high that if you head into the lower regions and keep at it, you will eventually find water.

*** 

# Find Insects

Pay close attention to prevalence of insects; place special attention on mosquito prevalence.

Most insects love to lay larvae in water pools and they also prefer to live close to water sources.

Mosquitoes will not be hard to spot, as they will actively seek you out. The more the insects, the higher the likelihood of a water source nearby.

***

# Find Damp Or Muddy Soil

If you find damp or muddy soil, dig into it. Digging into it may unearth an underground source of water.

This should be your last option; underground water is very rarely clean or fit for immediate consumption.

However, even dirty water will help you survive.
It is best to use your hands to dig, as unlike sticks and rocks, they will actually scoop dirt off the hole.

***

## Collect Rainwater

If it rains, make sure to collect rainwater; it is fit for immediate consumption. You can cup your hands, use a container, leaves, or just about anything you can get to collect water.

***

After getting water, it is recommended that you prepare it for consumption. Let's learn more about that next.

# 6. HOW TO PURIFY WATER

Since you cannot carry large amounts of water around without hampering your progress, it is important to understand how to purify the water you find in the wilderness.

These are the four most important water purification methods:

1. Filtering
2. Boiling
3. Chemicals
4. Solar Energy

*** 

## Filtering

For starters, it is a bit foolish to bother lugging manufactured filters around in the wilderness. The problem with them is that they are complex, heavy and expensive things.

It is always a good idea to filter your water before you do anything with it, including boiling. A t-shirt or a sock will do the job of removing gunk. However, paper coffee filter is the best material to use for simple filtering. It is also very light to carry around.

***

## Boiling

This is the best way to eradicate bacteria and viruses in your water. Make sure to bring it to a proper, roiling boil and let it hold for a full minute. While a metal canteen or pot is best, you can easily boil water in bark or plastic. The idea is to be careful, making sure that your container is not too close so it doesn't burn or melt.

***

## Chemicals

Carrying a couple of bottles of tincture iodine 2% will not be too much of a hassle. The most effective way to purify your water is to add a couple of drops of this to your water container.

Keep it simple; forego the small purification pills (which contain nothing more than tincture of iodine anyway) as they do not last as long as a bottle of the same. If this is not an option, bleach will do the job too. Just add in several drops and shake thoroughly.

***

38

## Solar Energy

If you have no other purifying means, leaving your clear water container in the sun for a day in sunny conditions, or two days in cloudy ones, will kill off bugs. This is done via UV radiation.

*** 

After you've collected and purified the water, then what? How do you preserve it? Let's learn that next!

# 7. HOW TO PRESERVE WATER

Once you have been able to purify your water, you will want to preserve at least a portion of it. You will want to be efficient with your time, and not have to purify water every time you feel like taking a sip.

These are a few ways that you can use to preserve purified water:

1. Commercial water bottles
2. Water barrels
3. Rain catchment systems

***

## Commercial Water Bottles

Plastic water bottles are light in nature and you can carry as many of them as possible. Simply wash these and refill them. Remember that they are designed to keep water so you can use these reliably. Here are a few facts:

41

- Many commercial water bottles are reusable at least once. Beyond this, plastic leaching may be a problem.

- Ordinary milk jugs are bad options. Not only do they not last as long as water bottles, they are also impossible to clean completely.

- 2-liter soda bottles are just as good. Just remember to disinfect before refilling.

*** 

## Water Barrels

55-gallon water barrels are not all that hard to lug around. They are great options for survivalists. They are usually blue and are made with solid plastic material. The best thing about them is that they can hold a lot of water.

*** 

## Rain Catchment Systems

These are basically systems you erect to collect and hold rainwater and runoff. They will serve you well as rainwater will be an option.

You can use all sorts of containers – from water barrels to soda bottles with the tops cut off. You will need funneling systems for maximum effectiveness, so do not discard the tops of soda bottles when you cut them off.

\*\*\*

So that's how you can preserve purified water. The next thing we will learn is how to make a fire, long before you start looking for food. Fire will be needed to boil water to make it fit for consumption, you can use fire to keep warm during cold weather, for signaling and for keeping off animals all this before you can have your first meal from the wilderness!

Let's learn how to make fire in the next chapter.

# 8. HOW TO MAKE A FIRE

It will be very difficult to survive long-term in the wild without being able to make fire. Fire not only provides warmth. It also allows you to cook animals and other food you hunted or found in the wild, while keeping big animals such as bears and wolfs away at night.

***

## What You Need To Make A Fire

Here are the things you need to make a fire:

1. Good fireplace
2. Firestarter
3. Tinder
4. Kindling
5. Fuel

***

**Good Fireplace**

Yes, you do need a proper fireplace if you are to make a proper fire. Select yours with care. Make sure your site is protected and sheltered from wind.

Also make sure there is a ready supply of fuel nearby (tinder and firewood).

Make sure to stay away from dry vegetation, which may catch fire and lead to a forest fire.

**Firestarter**

To start a fire, you will need to create that first spark or flame. For this reason, it will be necessary to stock up fire starters (see Chapter 3 'How To Prepare Your Survival Kit'), lighters and even matches. These will make it easier to light fires.

If you forget, or run out of fire starters, you will learn below how to start a fire without them.

**Tinder**

Tinder is material that lights easily. The best tinder is dry material that will only need a spark to light up. Your tinder must be thoroughly dry. You can use paper, grass, leaves, bark and resin as tinder. Resin also burns when wet, making it extremely good tinder. You will use tinder to start fires.

**Kindling**

This is material that is readily combustible. You will need to add this to already burning tinder. Small twigs are usually best for kindling.

Good kindling lights easily as long as there is a small flame going. Dead branches also provide good kindling.

**Fuel**

Find bigger pieces of wood that you can use to keep your fire going. It is crucial that all your woods are dry: it will smoke instead of burn if it is wet. You will need a good balance between softwood and hardwood. Softwood is best for getting your fire started, but hardwood will burn much longer and give off much more heat.

\*\*\*

## How To Make A Fire With A Lighter

Once you have everything in place, you are ready to make a fire.

47

Here is how to do it:

- Prepare building your fire by putting the tinder and kindling on the ground.

- Place some softwood over it, and then add hardwood.

- Begin your fire with lighting the tinder.

- Once you have your first flames, turn it into a fire by adding oxygen. You can use a fan, or even blow on it. Apply moderation though; you don't want to blow out the fire!

- Keep the fire going by adding more hardwood to it.

***

## How To Make a Fire Without Matches Or A Lighter

Suppose you forget matches, lighter or another fire starter, or simply run out? How can you make a fire then?

There are several ways you can light a fire without matches. However, making a fire using flint and steel has to be one of the more efficient ones.

Here is how to make a fire using flint and steel:

- Grip your rock and a piece of birch or fungus (basically tinder).

- Hold a piece of rock between thumb and forefinger and make sure there is a two-inch edge hanging out.

- Proceed to grasp your fungus between thumb and flint.

- Strike! Strike the steel against your flint several times. Sparks will fly off and land on your tinder, leading to a glow.

- Start your fire. Gently blow on your smoldering tinder to start it.

- To further build your fire, see the instructions above on how to build a fire with a lighter.

So that is how you build a fire if you don't have matches or a lighter.

You should ensure you carry a good flint and steel set, along with the matches, fire-starters and lighters. While matches may get wet and be useless and while lighter fluid eventually gets used up, a flint and steel set is perpetual. And you can always get a spark from striking steel against flint.

If you do not have a flint and steel set, it is easy to improvise. Simply use quartzite and your pocket knife's steel blade. Or try a magnifying glass and direct the sun's rays to start your fire!

***

Now that you know how to build a fire, let's move on and learn about how to find food in the wilderness.

# 9. HOW TO FIND FOOD

You can last in the wild without food for a couple of weeks. Much longer than you can without water.

However, lacking food can have severe consequences on your mental as well as physical health. Spending a few days without food decreases your energy levels; thereby slowing down your mental function. With less focus and low energy, it will be more difficult to find food, thus creating a vicious circle. So make finding food a priority!

If you apply the following strategies set out in this chapter, you won't have to starve in the wilderness:

- Prepare By Stocking Foods

- Foraging For Food

- Hunting And Setting Traps

- Gardening

***

# Prepare By Stocking Foods

Here are some key foods that you will be wise to stock up for survival in the wilderness:

- Unsweetened cocoa powder

- Crackers Dried legumes (beans, lentils, peas)

- Peanut butter

- Pasta sauce

- Flour (white, whole wheat)

- Sugar Canned fruits, vegetables, meats, and soups

- Whole grains (bulgur, barley, couscous, cornmeal, quinoa, oats, rice, wheat)

- Bouillon cubes or granules (vegetable, chicken, beef)

- Kitchen staples (baking powder, baking soda, yeast, vinegar)

- Honey

- Seeds (for eating and sprouting)

- Jell-O, pudding mixes

- Nonfat dried milk

- Popcorn (not the microwavable kind)

- Plant-based oil (corn oil, vegetable oil, coconut oil, olive oil)

- Cereals

- Packaged meals (hamburger helper, macaroni and cheese, Ramen noodles, etc.)

- Instant potato flakes

- Purified drinking water

If you want to learn more about what foods to stockpile in preparation for when an attack or disaster changes life as you know it, check out my other book: 'SHTF Prepping: The Proven Insider Secrets For Survival, Doomsday and Disaster Preparedness'.

But this book is about survival. So the question is: how do

you find food in the wilderness when your supplies are depleted?

* * *

# Foraging For Food

Here are a few insider tips for foraging in the wilderness:

1. Stay close to home
2. Stay away from large scale farming areas
3. Keep it simple
4. Do not gorge on wild plants
5. Examples of foods to find in the wilderness

## Stay Close To Home

For as long as you can, stay close to home and concentrate your foraging efforts on areas around home. Why is this?

Well, those wild plants, which usually grow closest to where people live are the plants, which are very best adapted to prop up your ability to survive, at least in that environment.

**Stay Away From Large Scale Farming Areas**

Stay away from areas that you know were once used as locations for large scale farming, even though they have since turned to wilderness. Why would this be recommended?

For one, large scale farming often comes with one large negative: wholesale spraying of herbicides and heavy use of chemical fertilizers.

Some of these chemicals take a long time before they get flushed off of the soil or the plants themselves and they are harmful.

**Keep It Simple**

Keep it simple for as long as you can.

Always go with the simple plants for as long as you can afford to, as it is harder to mistake these for other plants that may be poisonous.

Take dandelions for instance; nobody will ever confuse any other plant for them and they make a great salad.

## Do Not Gorge On Wild Plants

Wild plants do not have the luxury of having fertilizers fed to the soil around their roots. They also do not have the luxury of having pesticides sprayed on them. Thus, they have to find natural ways of surviving. This also means that a lot of them are very potent.

If you introduce large amounts too soon to your body, a negative reaction may result. Therefore, always eat small amounts at a time.

## Examples Of Foods To Find In The Wilderness

Here are several simple foraging options that work perfectly:

- Acorns. Dry them out, grind and rinse acids out

- Pine needles

- Pine cone nuts

- Weeds like fox tail, plantain. Dry and grind

- Water weeds, for example coon tail, reeds, wild rice and arrowhead

- Maple and Birch tree sap

- Frogs, turtles

- Clams and crayfish

These are just a few examples of what you can find in the wilderness.

If you really want to prepare yourself for what it is like to survive in the wild, your best bet is to find a guide and explore the wilderness together. Going out in the field with an experienced mentor will be your best possible training. Finding the edible plants, understanding which ones are poisonous. These are best learned under supervision.

Alternatively, if you can't find a teacher, buy a couple of books on foraging. Pick books that contain a lot of images and illustrations. These will be most helpful when learning to understand what plants can help you survive, and which don't.

***

## Hunting And Setting Traps

Hunting game on dry land often takes effort. While spears, slingshots and arrows do work, they often require strain and quite a bit of training. There are better hunting methods, such as:

1. Noosing
2. Setting traps

**Noosing**

Try using noosing wands to catch small game like fowl or rabbit.

A noosing wand is easy to set up:

- You only need a length of rope and a wand, such as a branch.

- Create a noose.

- Stretch the other rope end all the way to the other wand end. This will allow you to tighten your noose at your liberty

It's that simple. The only trouble with noosing is that you have to exercise extreme patience as you wait and even then, fast small game will run before you can close the noose around them.

## Setting Traps

Traps are often the best option. Pit traps will only be effective in some situations.

Here is how you create a pit trap:

- Dig a pit that is large enough to hold the animal you are targeting.

- Disguise the hole and wait for an animal to fall in.

- Consider putting spikes at the pit bottom. You can even put water in the hole to make life harder for the animal.

Your best option will be setting up many small snare traps to catch small game like raccoons and squirrels.

If you want to hit the jackpot often, set your trap near a game trail, or a water source where animals regularly come to drink.

***

# Gardening

Ultimately, you want to start growing your own food, instead of depending solely on food found in the wild. To do so effectively, it is important to learn as much as you can about gardening. You should know seasonal performance of crops. Learn the basics of crop husbandry and how to be self-reliant.

You don't need to know everything about gardening, but a few things can be quite helpful, like sprouting.

You can sprout grains like wheat, millet, rice, rye and corn. Legumes like mung beans, lentils, soybeans, garbanzo beans and black beans are also good for sprouting. Likewise, cabbage, onion, and broccoli are some of the vegetables that you can sprout. All these can be sourced from your local store's produce section.

To sprout, do the following:

- Look for sprouting trays or quart jars. You can improvise if possible. Get the sprouting seeds too.

- Put the seeds in a jar. The jar should have a lid that contains drainage holes. You can improvise the jar lid by punching some holes in any metallic lid.

- Pour water into the jar to the bream and rinse the seeds before draining them through the lid.

- Refill the jar with water and leave the seeds to soak overnight.

- The next day, drain the water from the jar and put the jar in a warm area (about 60-80 degrees Fahrenheit), away from direct sunlight. Keep rinsing them twice daily while draining excess water. The sprouts should start growing; within 3 to 5 days, your sprouts should have matured for consumption.

- Once the sprouts start maturing, expose them to sunlight. You can put your sprouts on a windowsill for a few hours to develop chlorophyll that defines sprouts' green coloring matter. Don't put the sprouts in direct sunlight.

- You can harvest and eat the sprouts after turning green.

You can eat sprouts while still raw as salads or after cooking them lightly. By sprouting legumes and grains, you have an opportunity to make an indoor garden whenever getting other fresh produce is difficult.

***

These are the basics of finding food in the wild. But as with water, you don't want to go foraging every time you start to feel hungry.

When you find food, you want to think ahead. Survival is all about building some reserves. So when you have been able to put your hands on some food, how do you preserve it? We will learn that next.

# 10. HOW TO PRESERVE FOOD

Now that you have a clear idea on how to find food in the wild, how do you preserve your food so that it sustains you for more than just one day?

How do you preserve your food so that it takes you beyond a week, maybe two?

\*\*\*

## The Basics Of Food Preservation

These are the basics of food preservation, both in the wilderness and in normal living:

- **Keep it frozen**. In the wilderness, if you can access ice, use it for freezing your food.

- **Keep it cool**. If you cannot freeze it, at least keep it cool. Foods kept at temps below 30 degrees Fahrenheit tend to outlast foods stored at higher temperatures.

- **Dehydrate it.** Dehydrating your foods will preserve them for much longer. This worked for our ancestors before the days of refrigeration. The sun and smoke come in handy in the wilderness.

***

## Keep It Frozen

Unless your shelter has electricity and you can power a fridge, freezing is pretty much only an option in the months of late fall and winter.

How do you freeze food in the wild?

- Use packed snow, or even ice you can cut from nearby ponds or lakes, to build an ice structure for your food.

- It will help to wrap your ice in wool or sawdust as this slows down melting.

Keep in mind that you need to clean your fish and game first, before freezing it for safe storage.

***

# Keep It Cool

When freezing food is not an option, at least keep it as cool as possible.

It will be necessary to keep your milk, meat supply and other fresh foods cool for days at a time, sometimes weeks.

DIY evaporation-based coolers will be useful in keeping your foods below 40 degrees Fahrenheit.

Here is how you can create a simple cooler:

- Obtain 2 vessels with porous material; plain wooden boxes and ceramic are great options. Make sure one vessel is small enough so it fits inside the other.

- Place filler between both vessels. Sponge and sand are great.

- Cover your inner vessel with a reflective surface, like a white towel, to deflect off heat easily.

- Use a hot location to pull water off the vessel as fast as possible.

- To replenish the water, simply pour it in at intervals.

***

# Dehydrate It

When summer is going on strong, sometimes cooling is not an option.

Dehydrating your foods is the next best option. You have two ways of going about this:

1. Sun drying
2. Smoke drying

## Sun Drying

The easiest and fastest way of meat and fish preservation is sun drying. Yet, you do not just dive in and dry your foods.

First of all, remove all bruised tissue, or tissue that looks infected. Wet fruit, fish and meat surfaces provide optimum conditions for bacteria. This is why drying is so effective – it gives bacteria very little chance.

Here is how to sun dry your foods:

- Cut your foods into thin strips.

- For fish and meat, cut 4-inch-wide strips and about 10 inches long and lay them on racks to dry.

- If you want to dry your food without necessarily cutting it up, skewer your fish or meat open and suspend it on a rope.

- You can sun dry your veggies and fruit by cutting them up into small sized pieces and laying them out in the sun.

**Smoke Drying**

If you have been able to make a fire, smoke drying is an excellent alternative to sun drying. Especially if the weather is cloudy, or flies and pests persist.

Here is how to smoke dry your foods:

- Build a fire.

- The fire does not have to be big: the purpose is to create smoke, not heat.

- The type of wood you use is important. Find hardwood, preferably still a bit green. You may even soak it if it is to try. Remember: you are trying to create smoke.

- Create an enclosure around the fire. This will keep the smoke in. You can use materials like a poncho, or parachute half. Make sure it does not come into contact with the fire.

- Now on to the meat or fish. As with sun drying, remove bruised and infected tissue first.

- Cut your meat or fish into strips here, about 2 inches (6 cm) thick. Put up a framework and drape the strips over them. Or simply skewer your food open and suspend it on smoking racks. Keep some distance between each strip, it is best if they do not touch.

- Place the food over the fire.

- During the smoking process, stay close to the fire and keep a close look at it. Make sure that the fire does not get too hot, and try to maintain a consistent temperature.

***

That is how you preserve food.

You now know how to keep your head cool in the wild, create a base camp, how to make a fire, how to find water and food, and how to preserve both.

With all of this in place, you will be able to survive in the wild for a long time.

However, the one thing that can threaten your survival is other people and wild animals. This means you ought to find ways of defending yourself when situation demands. We will learn how to go about that next.

# 11. HOW TO DEFEND YOURSELF

It is a good thing to learn how to use a firearm. It is an even better thing to carry one with you in the wilderness as it greatly increases your chances of survival.

However, as you may have watched in just about every SHTF (which stands for Shit Hits The Fan) based movie, ammunition is apt to become scarce. For this reason, you will have to learn to defend yourself without firearms; to improvise and respond appropriately to attacks.

So your ammo is over? You have no gun?

Breathe easy; this chapter will teach you a few self-defense techniques that require no firearms.

We will discuss two things:

- Improvise your weaponry

- Master a few hands-on self-defense techniques

Mastering these two can mean the difference between life and death in a threatening situation.

\*\*\*

## Improvise Your Weaponry

In order to protect yourself in the wild, be it against big animals like bears or wolves, or against other people trying to take away your shelter and food, you will need to have some sort of weapon.

And you will also need weapons to find that food in the first place.

The more weapons you have, the bigger your chance of hunting and defending yourself and your loved ones successfully.

Here are some basic weapons you can make and use in the wild:

- **Club**: Clubs have been around since man picked up a fallen branch and thought to use it as a weapon.

    Well, there are steps you can take to ensure your club serves you better.

For starters, dead, fallen branches make poor clubs. This is because they may be rotten. Select a wood piece from a living tree if you have time before an encounter. As a rule, your limb should not be thicker than an inch or so. Make sure it is as straight as can be and no longer than 5 feet.

- **Rocks**: This is the most basic of weaponry. By virtue of its mass alone, a rock will impart a lot of energy into a target.

  Consider this: a one-pound rock will easily crack a rib or even a skull when thrown by an adult of average strength. This is something that mere fists and feet cannot do.

  If you have the time, select the smoothest possible rock.

- **War Club**: This is a stick and stone combination.

  You will split one end of the stick in half and extend the slice to around 8 inches. The next step is to insert a one-pound rock within and then lash the whole thing together with a shoelace.

  What you finally have is a weapon that is extremely

capable of shattering a skull or breaking a set of adult ribs in several places.

***

# Master A Few Hands-On Self-Defense Techniques

There may be times when you need to defend yourself barehanded. You are caught by surprise, or for whatever reason don't have access to your weaponry.

In that case, you will need to rely on hands-on self-defense techniques.

Here are two of the most common attacks on people and how you can maneuver out of them:

- **The Front And Back Choke**: What is the first impulse you have when someone grabs you in a choke-hold?

  Usually, you will attempt to remove the choking-arm from around your neck. You will not be able to, though, as his arm is well positioned to stay locked.

  What you do here is you literally place your hand on his esophagus behind you and squeeze as hard as possible while attempting to work your way out of his

74

hold. This combination of activities will put your attacker off.

- **Defending Against The Bear Hug**: This hold will see your attacker grabbing your body and arms from behind in a tight grip.

  If you can, stomp him as hard as you can. High heels help, though it makes no sense as to why you would have high heels off the grid.

  The other thing to do is to slam his head using your elbows repeatedly.

To prepare for defending yourself in the wild, do not solely depend on reading these techniques. You will want to practice, to the extent where you can act on autopilot in case of a threat. When someone is attacking you, you do not have time to open this book and reread how to defend yourself. You don't even have time to think. You need to act immediately!

Therefore, practice, practice, and practice some more. The best thing you can do is actually follow some self-defense classes. This way, you can practice the techniques with other people, and mimic a possible attack.

\*\*\*

That is how you can defend yourself when you are faced with a threat.

Regardless of how much you prepare though, chances are you will still get hurt when attacked in the wild. In that case, having first aid skills can make your life a lot smoother. Let's learn some of those next.

# 12. HOW TO APPLY FIRST AID

When you are injured or getting sick in the wild, you will likely not be able to visit a doctor and get medical treatment. You won't even be able to get over-the-counter medicines.

The most basic first-aid equipment can save your life when your health is affected.

Let's look at:

- First Aid Basics

- Preparing Your First Aid Kit

- Maintain A Survivor's Mindset

\*\*\*

## First Aid Basics

Here are the basics of giving first aid in the following situations:

- Controlling the bleeding

- Caring for shock

- Caring for burns

- Caring for muscle, bone and joint injuries

- Caring for poisoning

**Controlling The Bleeding**

Cuts are the most common injuries, especially when living in the wilderness.

What do you do?

- Start with covering the wound with dressing

- Apply direct pressure against the wound

- Raise the injured area above heart level if there are no broken bones

- Then cover the dressing with a bandage

- If the bleeding is not stemmed by this, keep applying additional dressings and bandages

- Press the artery against the bone using a pressure point

**Caring For Shock**

Shock is a medical condition that can be life threatening. It can occur when a person is severely ill or injured.

To help a person who is in shock:

- Make sure the victim does not stay in too much heat or too much cold

- Raise the legs about one foot high if there are no broken bones

- Absolutely do not give him any food or drink

**Caring For Burns**

Burns can be caused by too much exposure to the sun or fire. They can also be the result of too much friction caused by carrying a heavy load for a long time, or simply from walking for too long.

Here is how you can reduce the pain caused by burns:

- Cool the burn gently

- Pour a lot of water on the burned area

- Cover with dry dressings

**Caring For Muscle, Bone And Joint Injuries**

If you are used to living a life of comfort, being out there in the wild can be tough. Your feet aren't used to all the sharp edges and surfaces from stones, twigs, and so on. Your legs aren't used to walking that much.

And even if you are prepared, life in the wild is rough. You may have to jump from one rock to another and make a miscalculation. Or a tree branch you are trying to hold on to breaks off.

Here is how you can treat muscle, bone and joint injuries:

- Rest the part with the injury

- Apply a cold pack, or ice if you can find some, to control the swelling

- Movement is a no-no here. If you must move the victim, immobilize the hurt part first

**Caring For Poisoning**

Poisoning can happen when you consume a plant or fungi that is not edible, or if you get bitten or stung by a venomous animal such as a snake or a scorpion.
Here is how you can deal with poisoning:

- If the victim has ingested poison, induce vomiting as this will help let some of the poison out.

- In case of a bite, apply a tight tourniquet above the bite area, swish some olive oil in your mouth and suck as much blood as you can from the wound while spitting it out.

- One of the greatest combat elements to poisoning is milk. Giving milk to the poisoned victim will often improve his situation.

\*\*\*

# The First Aid Kit

To amplify your survival chances in the wild, it is necessary to assemble a first aid kit and carry it with you. You can bet that at some point, you will get hurt or catch illness. To remedy the situation, it is necessary to prepare for survival by stocking up personal medication.

You can buy prepackaged first aid kits at most convenience stores. Alternatively, you can also assemble a proper first aid kit yourself.

Here is what the American Red Cross recommends you include in a first aid kit:

- 2 absorbent compress dressings (5 x 9 inches)

- 25 adhesive bandages (assorted sizes)

- 1 adhesive cloth tape (10 yards x 1 inch)

- 5 antibiotic ointment packets (approximately 1 gram)

- 5 antiseptic wipe packets

- 2 packets of aspirin (81 mg each)

- 1 blanket (space blanket)

- 1 breathing barrier (with one-way valve)

- 1 instant cold compress

- 2 pair of non-latex gloves (size: large)

- 2 hydrocortisone ointment packets (approximately 1 gram each)

- scissors

- 1 roller bandage (3 inches wide)

- 1 roller bandage (4 inches wide)

- 5 sterile gauze pads (3 x 3 inches)

- 5 sterile gauze pads (4 x 4 inches)

- oral thermometer (non-mercury/non-glass)

- 2 triangular bandages

- tweezers

Make sure you to check if any prepackaged first aid kit includes these items. If not, buy the missing items separately and add them to your kit.

Visit **redcross.org** for more information.

***

## Maintain A Survivor's Mindset

This is the most important of all perhaps. If your mind "breaks" and you lose control over yourself, you will die soon enough. With a healthy state of mind, you can live on only the most essential of things, improvising along as you move.

Without a sound mind, you can have the best of equipment and yet be unable to use any of it to help your survival. In the beginning of this book, we spoke of the importance of embracing a survivor's mindset.

Remember Poon Lim? He survived for 133 days in the sea on a small makeshift raft. He was exposed to the hot sun every day, and constantly on the verge of starvation and dehydration. He used a sharpened piece of metal as a knife. And he drank the blood of sea gulls to stay hydrated, because even though he was surrounded by water, it wasn't drinkable.

He had the survivor's mindset. It is this mindset that allowed him to endure these barbaric circumstances and stay alive until he was finally rescued.

A survivor's mindset will give you the necessary mettle to persevere and maintain sound mental health. Without a survivor's mindset, survival becomes almost unviable.

So regardless of your external circumstances, always check in with your mindset and be vigilant in keeping your hopes up high. It will be the fuel that keeps you going when all hope may seem lost.

# FINAL WORDS

Thank you for picking up a copy of this book, and sticking around all the way to the end. I'm impressed: this tells me you are taking Survival seriously, and are willing to adopt a survivor's mindset!

I hope this book was able to help you to understand how to survive anywhere.

This book is all about keeping things simple and making forward steps off the grid. You may have caught perhaps the biggest hint of all: you will have to be open to **improvisation**.

For what is survival if not constantly improvising and adapting to conditions so you fit your circumstances better?

The next step is to implement what you have learned: a smart person is prepared for any situation, even though he hopes for the best.

# BONUS CHAPTER: INTRODUCTION TO SHTF PREPPING

If you enjoyed in this book, you may also be interested in my other book: '**SHTF PREPPING:** *The Proven Insider Secrets For Survival, Doomsday and Disaster Preparedness*'

Below is a chapter of that book: '*Introduction to SHTF Prepping.*'

It is my way of saying thanks for:

- [ ] reading this book, and
- [ ] taking survival seriously. You rock!

Let's get started, shall we?

*\*\*\**

# Natural Disasters

To say we live in uncertain times would be an understatement.

In 2020, the coronavirus pandemic shook the world. Schools, restaurants and office buildings were closed. Also, basic human rights (such as freedom of movement) were restricted. At the time of writing, it is unclear how long it will take before effective medication is available. It is expected that the it will take years for the world economy to fully recover.

Unfortunately, the coronavirus pandemic isn't unique. There were many other disasters in recent years. Regardless of whether you believe in global warming or not, you can't deny the devastating effects of the natural disasters that have shaken the world recently. When hurricanes Katrina (2005), Sandy (2012) and Michael (2018) hit the coast, they killed almost two thousand people combined. Moreover, many more people were injured, their homes ruined. Cities were flooded, infrastructure was destroyed.

2004 saw one of the deadliest natural disasters recorded in history. An earthquake in the Indian Ocean with a moment magnitude of 9.1-9.3 triggered multiple tsunamis killing between 230,000 and 280,000 people in fourteen countries, mostly in Asia.

And in 2011, an earthquake followed by a tsunami led to the Fukushima Daiichi nuclear disaster in Japan. The tsunami destroyed the emergency generators that provided power to cool the reactors, resulting in three nuclear meltdowns and the release of radioactive material.

Finally, the 2018 California wildfires has had a devastating impact on the lives of thousands of Americans.

***

## Terrorist Attacks

Also, in the last few decades, terrorist attacks have become more and more prevalent. Where at first 9/11 seemed to be a (major) isolated incident, terrorist attacks have now become much more common. Some recent examples are:

- Madrid train bombings (2004), where ten bomb explosions aboard Cercanías commuter trains killed 192 civilians.
- London train bombings (2005), where a series of suicide bombs went off in London's underground trains and a double-decker bus, killing 52 civilians.
- Charlie Hebdo shooting (2015), where two terrorists killed 12 people in the offices of the French satirical weekly newspaper Charlie Hebdo.

- Bangkok bombing (2015), where 20 civilians were killed at the Erawan Shrine.
- Paris attacks (2015), where a number of terrorists started shooting and blew up bombs at a number of locations, including the area just outside the Stade de France in Saint-Denis during the soccer game between France and Germany, and the Bataclan theatre, where Eagles of Death Metal were playing a gig. 130 civilians were killed.
- Brussels airport and train station bombings (2016), where two suicide bombers at Brussels Airport and one at Maalbeek metro station killed 32 civilians.
- Nice attack (2016), where a truck drove into crowds celebrating Bastille Day, killing 86 civilians.
- Berlin attack (2016), where a truck drove into a Christmas market, killing 12 civilians.
- Barcelona attack (2017), where a vehicle hit pedestrians in Las Ramblas, killing 15 civilians.

The threat and unpredictability of these terrorist attacks instill great fear in many people, while at the same time bringing a Big Brother government as described by George Orwell in his classic novel '1984' closer and closer.

In 2013, Edward Snowden, a former CIA employee, revealed classified documents showing how the National Security

Agency (NSA) tapped anyone and everyone, even heads of foreign states, in their hunger for information.

And in February 2017, China made it mandatory for all car owners in the Bayingolin prefecture in the Xinjiang region to install a GPS system in their vehicle. By being able to track where all cars are at any time, the government hopes to prevent terrorist attacks. Vehicle owners who refuse to install the system will no longer be able to refuel at gas stations.

\*\*\*

## Inequality In Wealth Distribution

The aftermath of the Great Recession, which started when Lehman Brothers filed for bankruptcy in September 2008, exposed a growing gap between the wealthy elite on the one hand, and the low and middle class on the other hand. In 2011, the Occupy movement coined the slogan 'We are the 99%', referring to a statistic that the top 1% wealthiest people have a disproportionate share of power and capital.

According to an analysis published by the National Bureau of Economic Research in December 2016, half of American adults have been *"completely shut off from economic growth since the 1970s."* Over that same period, the income skyrocketed for the top one percent.

When running for president of the United States, Donald Trump was able to capitalize on this sentiment with his 'Make America Great Again' campaign, which ultimately got him elected. However, his tendency to act mostly on impulse, his disliking of immigrants, and his dismissal of any news that he doesn't like as 'fake news', are not the best indicators for political stability during his presidency. It may in fact even hasten a collapse of respect for government institutions.

\*\*\*

## NOW Is The Time For SHTF Prepping

In light of all these recent developments, a disaster is not just something that you can see in movies such as 'Deep Impact', 'The Book of Eli' and 'Mad Max', while leaning back in a comfortable, cushioned chair, snacking on popcorn and sipping on a coke.

What you see in these movies may soon be a reality. And now is the time to prep for it!

Like the biblical Joseph, who helped prepare Egypt for seven years of famine following seven years of abundance, don't be blinded by your current level of comfort. Think ahead now, and you will thank yourself later.

Many people are already aware of the urgency. For example, when National Geographic Channel's reality show 'Doomsday Preppers' premiered in 2012, a whopping four million viewers were watching, and later on it became the most popular show in the channel's history. The show focused on people prepping for SHTF.

And perhaps even more importantly: the elite are already prepping for SHTF! In the article 'Doomsday Prep For The Super-Rich', published in 2017 in The New Yorker, a number of them confirmed they are prepping for disasters:

- **Steve Huffman (co-founder and C.E.O. of Reddit)**: underwent laser eye surgery to improve his chances of surviving in case SHTF.
- **Antonio García Martínez (former Facebook product manager)**: bought five wooded acres on an island. He also bought solar panels, generators, as well as ammunition, and shipped it to the island.
- **A head of an investment firm**: has a helicopter gassed up all the time. He also has an underground bunker equipped with an air-filtration system.
- **Larry Hall**: developed the Survival Condo Project. This is a luxury apartment complex with fifteen stories. It is built in an underground Atlas missile silo. It has twelve private apartments that were advertised for three million dollars. Each unit has been sold.

Disasters can happen at any time, disrupting and endangering your life and that of your loved ones. When they hit, they strike fast. If you wait until then to build a shelter, stock on supplies and learn new skills, it will be too late.

By contrast, being prepared for such catastrophic events gives you confidence to face emerging challenges and you are likely to pick up the pieces quickly.

The trick lies in knowing what to do and when to do it.

And you have come to the right place!

In this book, you will learn all the ins and outs of SHTF prepping. You will get the best ideas, skills and knowledge to hold onto as you take full control of your life irrespective of what nature or your fellow men throw at you!

Are you ready?

***

*This is the end of this bonus chapter.*

*Want to continue reading?*

*Then get your copy of "SHTF Prepping" at your favorite bookstore!*

# DID YOU LIKE THIS BOOK?

If you enjoyed this book, I would like to ask you for a favor.

Would you be kind enough to share your thoughts and post a review of this book? Just a few sentences would already be really helpful.

Reviews are the lifeblood of independent authors. I know, you're short on time. But I would really appreciate even just a few sentences!

Your voice is important for this book to reach as many people as possible.

The more reviews this book gets, the more people will be able to find it and learn how they can survive outdoors.

\*\*\*

IF YOU DID NOT LIKE THIS BOOK, THEN PLEASE TELL ME! You can email me at **feedback@semsoli.com**, to share with me what you did not like!

Perhaps I can change it.

A book does not have to be stagnant, in today's world. With feedback from readers like yourself, I can improve the book. So, you can impact the quality of this book, and I welcome your feedback. Help make this book better for everyone.

Thank you again for reading this book and good luck with applying everything you have learned!

I'm rooting for you...

# ABOUT THE AUTHOR

Gavin Williams lives in Leavenworth, with his wife, two sons and their dog (an Irish wolfhound).

He loves to explore the outdoors, often with his dog. Surviving in the wilderness, going back to the essence of what it means to be a man, is what makes him tick.

From a very young age, when his father would take him out camping in the wilderness, he learned how to survive with the bare minimum. He knows how to make a shelter from only natural materials, how to read animal trails to find food and water, how to make a fire. And he wants to share his expertise.

That's why Gavin authored multiple books on surviving outdoors. And more books are coming, so keep a lookout for that!

# BY THE SAME AUTHOR

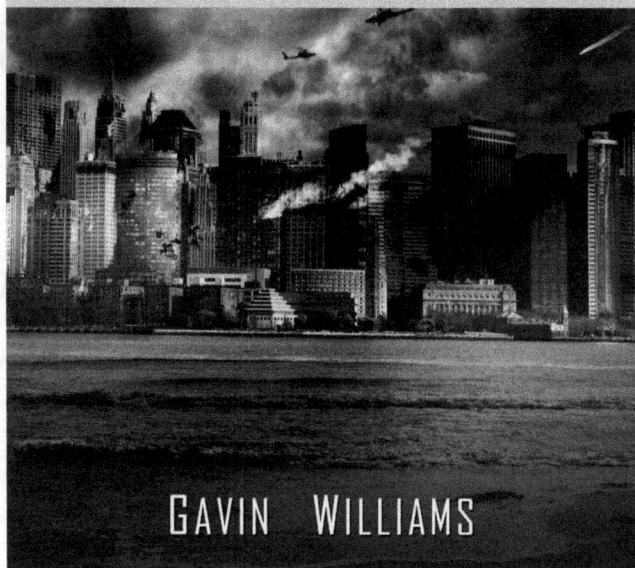

SHTF PREPPING

THE PROVEN INSIDER SECRETS FOR SURVIVAL, DOOMSDAY AND DISASTER PREPAREDNESS

GAVIN WILLIAMS

# NOTES